How to Lose Weight Eating Out

A Guide to Navigate Restaurant Menus

I0434839

Nate Gration

www.theonlinetrainers.com

Acknowledgements

To God who leads and guides my path each day.

To my family and wife who are always there with a supporting hand.

To my clients at Lasseters Health Club who are an inspiration.

To my work colleagues Matt, Alexandra, and the extended Lasseters Team who encourage personal development and betterment.

Introduction

I want to thank you and congratulate you for downloading the book, "*How To Lose Weight Eating Out: A Guide To Navigate Restaurant Menus*".

This book contains proven steps and strategies on how to enjoy eating out without compromising your diet.

The journey to weight loss is never easy as it calls for a complete lifestyle shift. Plenty of sacrifices are in order for those who are trying their best to diet and keep fit.

Apart from adopting a regular workout schedule and foregoing a sedentary lifestyle, it's also necessary that a healthier eating regimen be considered.

Healthy means cutting back on the junk and focusing more on good meals, day in and day out.

What worries most dieters is the misconception that they have to stop eating out if they want to lose weight. These days, when almost everyone prefers eating out than staying in and cooking, not eating out every now and then is not really as feasible and sustainable as it used to be.

In addition, having too many restrictions can discourage someone from continuing their attempt at being healthy, especially with tons of temptations and distractions surrounding them.

It's not easy being on a diet. And regardless of its rewards, it's something that can easily put a damper on the way food is enjoyed. In a restaurant setting, navigating the menu can be a stressful process indeed but, it's not impossible to find food you can work with even in a fast food environment.

There are a number of tricks, tips, and practices that you will learn of in this book that will help you navigate menus effectively; helping you continue with your weight loss journey even if eating out is part of your daily, weekly, or monthly regimen.

Remember that we're not here to tell you what to eat when you dine out. We're here to teach you how to go about menu offerings so that regardless of where you choose to dine in, you'll be able to find the best options to go with without feeling deprived.

Read and understand the tips provided in this book and you won't feel as if you're dieting the next time you eat out. You'll also be surprised at how much more satisfying eating out will be without the consequence of added poundage.

It's good advice to take things slow and figure out what works best given the weight loss plan you are currently engaged in. If there are certain restrictions in your diet (like reducing salt, sugar, or avoiding certain ingredients) as provided by your nutritionist then feel free to include those as you apply the practices that will be discussed in this book.

Keep in mind that the practices here are not universal. Some will work better for others and some may not. This is why it would be best if you work to thoroughly understand everything before applying the concepts to your daily dining routine. Also make it a point to take note of your progress and weigh out the best practices for your needs.

Thanks again for downloading this book, I hope you enjoy it!

information is without contract or any type of guarantee assurance.

The trademarks that are used are without any consent, and the publication of the trademark is without permission or backing by the trademark owner. All trademarks and brands within this book are for clarifying purposes only and are the owned by the owners themselves, not affiliated with this document.

Chapter 1 Eating Out – What's the Problem?

The reality for most people is that instead of staying at home, they choose to go out and eat in their restaurants of choice. On average, people leisurely eat out as much as four times a week, and this does not include eating out during lunchtime at the office.

Not only is eating out easy, but there are cases when it's more affordable compared with the costs of preparing food at home (if you include the time spent shopping and prepping). And when it comes to people who lead fast-paced lifestyles, frequently eating out becomes the norm.

People eat out for a number of reasons. For one, it's a common practice during the workday. Next, it's a fun leisure activity. Third, not having to prep meals can be a huge lifesaver if you don't know how to cook or if you're simply too tired to cook. When you choose to eat out, you order, eat, pay, and that is about it -- there's no muss, no fuss, and absolutely no hassle.

In general, eating out shouldn't be as complicated as some of us make it out to be. But there are people who can just order anything out of the menu while the rest have to look through every item, description, and assess whether or not this meal is ideal given the diet plan that they have currently embraced. The problem in this case is not eating out per se but knowing how to order when you do.

Chapter 2 Put the Fun Back in Eating Out -- The Solution

Eating should be a fun activity whether or not you are dieting and every chance that you get to eat out should be a treat in itself, whether you are with loved ones or even by yourself.

If you are trying to lose weight, don't see it as a detriment to enjoying food. Instead, learn about how best to navigate menus so that you can enjoy delicious food when you decide to dine out.

There are a number of things that you have to consider when eating out and here are some of them. Take things slow and understand how to approach these when you see them in the menu. For the rest, embrace them as regular practices and apply them to your lifestyle.

The great thing about the tips that you will read about shortly is that you can also apply them to your home-cooking methods, mindset, and attitude. These will help you shift the way you think about food and make those diet and weight loss goals of yours much easier to attain, not to mention sustain.

- Beverages
  More often than not, when you go out to eat, you'll notice that a number of restaurants will start you off with some beverages. For someone who is dieting, the main advice that's commonly given is to stick with plain old water. But there are instances when water may not cut it. And when you find yourself in a restaurant, apart from navigating the food menu, you might also have to navigate the beverage menu.

There are plenty of people who share the same sentiment wherein they feel that the beverage menu is more complicated than the one for food. This is because most of the time, there are simply far too many drinks to choose from.

A standard beverage menu in a mid to high-class restaurant can be as lengthy as a standard food menu and through the pages, you'll find listings including everything from your typical sodas and juices to your list of wines from around the world.

So if you're on a diet and would like to partake in a beverage other than water during your meal out, narrow down your beverage choices. First, steer clear of the water list. If you're not having service water, then there's no sense in paying more for bottled water (unless necessary) -- one down and a gazillion to go.

The next step is to skip beverages that are high in sugar. This means sodas and juices, unless the latter means fresh-squeezed. Chances are the beverage list will be categorized so this task will not be as tedious as it seems. This will leave you with fresh-squeezed juices, wines, coffees, teas, and other alcoholic offerings (on most occasions). Black coffee and tea (with or without honey) are excellent choices to end a meal with. Wines are excellent to have during the meal. As for juices, they can go before, during, or after the meal.

Fruits are friends for dieters so your choices won't be as limited here. Just make sure that you check the menu or ask the waiter about any added sugar. You can ask them to prepare your drink without it.

As for wines, steer clear of wine cocktails and instead go for wines in bottles. You'll find these stated clearly on the menu. You can choose to go by the glass or, if you're with company, by the bottle. But remember to limit your consumption to about a glass serving's worth.

As for other alcoholic offerings, only set your eyes on the pure alcohol like vodka, gin, or even tequila and have yourself a shot. Other drinks like cocktails and the like should be avoided as these usually come with other ingredients (and sugar) mixed in.

Now that you know how to narrow down a beverage menu, you won't encounter as many issues the next time you're exposed to a lengthy list. Using the available categories printed on the pages, you can easily find the kinds of drinks that will do your diet good and still enable you to lose weight even if you eat out.

- Soups and Salads

What do you find at the beginning of a menu? Usually, you'll be greeted by a selection of soups and salads together with appetizers on one page. The thing about soups and salads is that they can both be diet-friendly or its mortal enemy.

Let's start with soups. The great thing about them is that they fill you up. This means that you'll have more chances of eating less later in your meal. Most of the time, people cut back on carbs and focus on proteins and this is a great way to eat healthily when you're out.

The problem with consuming soup is not choosing the right one to order. In a restaurant, you'll have two styles of soup; something with a flavorful broth or something that's filled to the brim with cream. If you choose the former, minestrone perhaps, you'll have something healthy, filling, and low on calories.

If you decide to order some cream of mushroom for example, the cream alone will fill you with an excess amount of fat. In this case, we're not talking about healthy and beneficial fats but those that easily make your love handles even easier to handle (if you catch my drift).

So when you eat out, decide if soup's something you just have to order. If you can skip it, by all means do (it will also save you a ton of money as soups, salads, and appetizers are usually priced relatively high for their worth). If you really want to have something warm to start your meal with, go for vegetable broths, consommés, and the like. Not only are these lighter but healthier as well. Provided that they are made from scratch, you'll get long-simmered soups packed with vitamins and minerals from vegetables and sometimes even lean meats.

As for the salad, don't be fooled by how healthy it can seem. Although it consists mainly of fresh greens and other vegetables, people are often blindsided by the dressing. There are plenty of salads that are loaded with heavy cream-style dressings laced with fat and sugar – unnecessary calories that lead to weight gain.

As you navigate the menu, check out what ingredients are being tossed in with the vegetables. If you see high-fat dressings, you can request that these be placed on the side. This way, you can control how much of it goes into your plate. For these creamy dressings, use a small dollop or measure out small amounts using your fork then spreading it onto the greens.

If you see ingredients like croutons, cheese, or bacon for example, it would be best if you chose another type of salad or have these placed on the side as well. Depending on your diet, you can forego these or measure out small amounts to add to your salad greens.

Depending on the restaurant that you dine in, some may offer options when it comes to dressings. In this case, go for lighter ones like vinaigrettes. You can also request this from the waiter. You also have the option of asking for some oil and lemon and making the dressing yourself. Just top it off with some salt and pepper.

Try to avoid starchy salads as well. Potato salad, macaroni, tuna and chicken salad, as well as coleslaw tend to come with a lot of mayo (fat) as well as sugar (added calories).

With these in mind, hopefully, you'll have an easier time working out the soup and salad section of the menu. It's not something you should stress over. You simply have to make a simple decision on whether or not to order these items, and if you do, make a selection on which ones make the most sense given that you are in the process of dieting.

- Others

  Apart from checking out the food items being offered, there are other things that you can take into consideration, plus additional practices that you can apply whenever you decide to eat out.

  As you will notice, these will come with some adjustment, effort, and getting used to but by taking the time to understand, adopt, and embrace them, you'll find it much easier to eat out, stick with your diet, and still lose weight while enjoying good food.

  * Know before you go

  Are you one of those people who love to research about destinations before you travel or look for product reviews before you go out and purchase something? Thanks to the Internet, doing your research when it comes to food and restaurants is easy as pie. Now there's no excuse for you not to do your research and know before you go.

  Apart from the World Wide Web, there are also countless mobile applications that cater to foodies around the world. You can get information from restaurant addresses and phone numbers to reviews and even have a full look at their menus and special offerings.

  This is why it's a good and smart practice, especially if you are dieting, to take a look at the place that you plan on visiting. Given that most, if not all restaurants are online these days, all it takes is a few clicks of a button for you to find their menus. So take the time to look these over. Most, if not all of their dishes will come with a description of the plate (cooking method and sometimes even seasonings and fat used included) so you can assess which ones are okay for your diet.

  It would be best if you went straight to the appetizers, salads, and grilled plates sections first. Usually, you will find enough options in these sections to make your scheduled dine out a feast to remember. Take note of the food items that interest you and make it a point to stick with these choices when you do visit the restaurant.

Check out drinks and dessert as well. For the latter, make it a habit to order some only if you still have room in your stomach after the end of the savory dishes. It's also a good idea to share a dessert instead of finishing an entire slice of cake, for example, by yourself.

Always remember that you taking the time to look menus over, ahead of your planned visit, can do wonders for your diet, not to mention your dining experience. For one, you won't be stressed to order out of impulse. Second, being aware of the quality and healthy-ness of your chosen dish will prevent any feelings of guilt or worry while you eat; hence a better overall dining experience.

It may sound simple but this kind of food planning is something that can really help you enjoy eating out while attempting to shed several pounds. And the more you do it, the more natural it will seem whenever you dine out in the future.

* Order first

So you've done your menu research. When you visit the restaurant, try your best to order first. This doesn't technically mean ordering your food while others are still checking out the available options. Simply put, it means being the first in your group to mention his or her chosen dish.

The rationale behind this is simple. In almost everything, we can get influenced by our peers to decide against ourselves, hence the term peer pressure. The same concept of peer pressure applies to ordering food in a restaurant.

Not that you'll be forced by a friend or relative to order something else on the menu, opposite a healthier choice you prefer. But their decision can also sway you to go towards the more indulgent route.

Say you're with a friend and most of them order steak and mash with heaping spoonfuls of gravy. Chances are, you'll eventually decide to order the same. But if you place your order first, you'll be all set. And chances are you won't be the kind of diner who will suddenly cancel everything and ask your waiter to change the meal that you specifically ordered.

But there may be instances when you can't be the first to order. If you find yourself in this position, simply close the menu (you know what you want anyway) and work from there. When it's your turn to place your order, simply repeat the dish that you've selected the night before as you were doing your menu rundown at home.

Should you find yourself in a restaurant that you frequent, it gets even easier as you don't need the menu at all. Usually we have that one favorite dish that we regularly order. If this is your healthy dish of choice then you can simply ask the waiter for your regular order. If you really frequent the establishment, they will know what you're talking about – special requests and all.

This should make it easier for you to dine out and not worry about messing up your diet. This will also prevent you from using the excuse that you gained weight because your friends or family asked you to eat out. Also, you wouldn't have to make the excuse of not attending the party because you are dieting. Again, all of the control will be in your court and dieting won't be a chore or restriction to your social life.

* Sit in a quiet area

If you think that the interior design of a restaurant serves no other purpose but satisfy aesthetic requirements then you are mistaken. Although the décor used in places like these serve to reflect the type of ambiance that's reflective of the cuisine being offered, it also serves to entice people to eat, eat, and eat.

For example, the use of certain colors alone can encourage, or rather influence people to keep on ordering food by stimulating their appetites. If you take notice, you'll realize that most food establishments - from grocery stores to restaurants and bars - have a fondness for using red in their décor. It can be used to paint the walls or as table accents (note the ever popular red checkered tablecloth). This is because red gets the job done; it indeed makes you hungrier.

Aside from red accents, you will find restaurants that have 2 distinct areas, one much quieter than the other. The latter is where you want to sit if you want to lose weight, eat healthy, and still have fun while you dine out with family or friends.

Unbeknownst to most people, sitting within the louder parts of a restaurant can influence or trigger excessive ordering. The areas in question include those near windows, TVs, or the bar area. The thing about it is that people have a tendency to eat more when there's a commotion in their midst.

As you're distracted by the noise, you tend to lose track of whatever it is that you've already consumed, from drinks to appetizers to mains and even that tempting breadbasket. As a result, you eat more, not to mention choose more unhealthy options than your diet permits.

Sitting in a quiet area also gives you and the people you're with a better time while you dine out because you'll be able to hear each other and engage in active conversation without the need to shout across the table. Now that's an automatic plus!

So the next time that you're making reservations, don't forget to make a headline for the quiet table in the establishment. Request it from the restaurant attendee and they'll gladly give you an available table. If you don't have a reservation, make the same request when you walk in. Should the restaurant be busy and have no available table at the moment when you arrive, choose to wait – it'll be well worth your time (and your diet will thank you).

* Change your dining mindset

As you navigate the menu, keep in mind that it's not just about reading what's there. To be able to choose healthier dishes and enjoy eating out while you diet, it's also necessary for you to alter your dining mindset. When it comes to this, here are several tips that can make a huge difference:

- Don't let certain words sway your decision

Just like how businesses utilize color and design to sway decisions and encourage sales, restaurateurs use similar tactics to encourage their diners to order more and choose food items that have higher profit margins.

This is precisely the reason why you should not let certain words sway your decision when eating out. Apart from saving you money, having more control in this department as you navigate menus will also help you stick with your diet regimen and weight loss routines.

For menus, customers are often enticed by amazing pictures of food accompanied by descriptions that are truly mouth-watering; you haven't ordered anything yet but the description itself is usually enough to make you salivate and crave for that particular item.

Remember that most menus are not created without any professional process. Descriptions are developed to have a certain effect on readers. Keywords like ripe, tender, juicy, legendary, velvety, and other adjectives that easily translate to tastes, textures, and sensations (what you'll supposedly feel when eating the dish) are what you need to be aware of.

By targeting your senses, you're most likely to be influenced to order certain dishes because your taste buds are somewhat prepped in a sense. Your mind is geared to think that you'll feel amazing when you indulge in these plates. Most of the time, restaurants deliver. But the food that comes with the promise may be problematic, given your diet.

If you want to lose weight and still be able to enjoy lunch or dinner out with family and friends, make sure to always have full control over your meal. Don't let these words sway you no matter what. Yes, it will take some getting used to (and a lot of will power as well). But simple sacrifices will do you (and your waistline) a lot of good.

- Don't think that mains are mandatory

Most of us have been geared to think that when eating out, we should get an appetizer, a main, and some dessert, but this is not the case. There's no rule stating that you should get several courses when you dine out and there's absolutely no rule stating that mains are mandatory.

When you eat out, you can still stick with your diet and lose weight if you change your mindset and stop thinking that the latter is so. There are lots of options for you to consider when you visit a restaurant.

When you view the menu, don't be fooled by the categories they use to separate dishes. If possible, remove them from the equation. Instead, focus on the dishes being served regardless of these labels.

You can get a salad or soup alone and call it a day. You can also choose to go with a supposed appetizer and only have that (because most of these come in serving sizes that are enough to fill you up just right).

So forget the notion that you need to order an entrée like lamb chops, pasta, or steak with mashed potatoes as you definitely don't have to; especially if you feel that they are overindulgent foods given your weight loss goals.

- Don't think that appetizers can't fill you up

It's common among diners to have this preconceived notion that appetizers are there to engage you for the upcoming entrée. But this is really not the case and by shifting your mindset, you can always eat out while dieting and still lose weight in the process.

Stop thinking that appetizers won't be enough to fill you up, as there are certain options that can serve as excellent entrée selections. Appetizers are tasty, and portion sizes enable you to order more than one type of dish and still not end up eating more than what your body needs.

Entrees usually come in hefty portions; sometimes excessive enough to feed two to three people. Appetizers on the other hand come in manageable portions.

The beauty of appetizers is that most restaurants also have a number of options that can be chosen from. You'll often find veggies, seafood, meat, and the like on the appetizer section alone. This means that you won't have to limit your options when you decide to order a small plate as an entrée.

But this doesn't mean that you have free reign over the appetizer list. It's still important that you look through what's available and go with healthier choices like those made with vegetables, seafood, or those that don't come with ingredients that are high in fat.

You can choose to combine two appetizers for your entrée or choose an appetizer and complementary broth soup or light salad. This way, you're sure to feel satisfied without all of the excess calories. You're able to eat out and still lose weight in the process, plus you can enjoy a multitude of flavors while you're at it – what's better than that?

So remember, appetizers are not only there to start your meal. They can fill you up and fast so don't limit yourself to the entrée section of the menu the next time you eat out.

- Don't think all desserts are bad

When dieting, one of the sections that anybody wants to skip (so as not to feel sad or deprived) is the dessert section. But don't think that all desserts are bad for you, or your diet as deprivation has a much worse effect overall.

When you read through the pages of your chosen restaurant's menu, don't hesitate to take a look at the desserts that they are offering. Consider the ingredients used and the type of dessert it is.

For example, try to avoid ice creams or gelatos and instead go with a sorbet or granita that are made without cream or eggs. If you see a cheesecake, maybe skip that and instead go with a healthier fruit assortment.

* Consider healthy swaps – have food prepared your way (don't be afraid to ask)

A lot of us make the mistake of thinking that restaurants can only serve whatever's written down on their menu. Especially these days when the food business is becoming more and more competitive, these establishments are working hard to satisfy every client that walks through their doors. This means that customization is something they welcome. In your case, this means that you can usually make special, but reasonable requests when you order out.

If you're unsure of a certain dish, ask your waiter about it before placing an order. Do the same if you are interested in a more indulgent dish that you're thinking twice about ordering. Not only will doing so get you more information about the food but you'll be able to asses whether or not your dietary concerns can be addressed.

Don't be afraid to ask questions and make any necessary requests but be respectful when you do. Here are some of the questions that you should consider asking if not already indicated:

- What ingredients are used to create this dish? Can I request to have a certain ingredient removed or substituted with a healthier alternative (then provide suggestions or ask for their recommendation)?

- What cooking method will you be using for this dish? Can the chef do this instead (grill, bake, broil, steam)?

- Which items on the menu are low in sugar, fat, or calories?

- What ingredient or sauce can I substitute for this (certain fats or oils, vegetables instead of starches or other carbohydrates, a leaner cut of meat perhaps)?

- How large is one serving of this dish? Can I ask you to split it for me (you can have one of the portions packed for another day – doggie bag)?

A number of restaurants accommodate special requests these days with more and more people becoming highly conscious of what they eat. You always have this option but make it a point not to force your requests upon the chef. Especially if they serve a particular type of cuisine, there may be certain ingredients that they just don't carry. You want them to be flexible and accommodate your needs but you have to be reasonable with your requests.

* 3-Bite Rule

Now, there are certain food items that your diet can do better without yet depriving yourself may cause more harm than good. When you find yourself in a situation where you'd like to try a more indulgent offering in the restaurant menu, follow what's known as the 3-Bite Rule.

The concept of the 3-Bite Rule is pretty simple. Take three bites of the not-so-healthy food, and with each one savor the flavor and experience, then walk away.

It'd be a good idea to share it with your co-diner but whatever happens, stay away from that plate after you'd indulged in your three portioned bites. Not only will this satisfy your craving but after some time, you won't even feel any inkling to have another go at it.

The great thing about the 3-Bite Rule is that it makes the entire process of navigating the menu a lot easier on your part. Since you'll have some leeway to indulge in something that's not as healthy as your main course, it won't take you such a long time to think, decide, and place your order.

* Be mindful of preparation

Most of us have the tendency of focusing too much attention on ingredients, thereby forgetting cooking methods and preparation as a result. If you want to lose weight without limiting yourself too much when you eat out, you should be mindful of prep as well.

It's really simple; the way your food is prepared plays a vital role when it comes to how much fat or how many calories you end up being served in a restaurant. So when you navigate a menu, make it a point to look for prep information. If this isn't provided, ask your waiter about it.

Although fried foods are tasty as can be, they are not the healthiest foods in the world. If you were dieting, it would be best if you stayed away or limited your consumption of fried foods (deep-fried, shallow-fried, or even pan-fried), which are often breaded (added carbohydrates) and dunked in oil (excess fat).

Look for these words instead: poached, baked, steamed, broiled, and grilled. All of these will give you equally-flavorful foods without the added calories. Usually, these cooking methods have the ability to help ingredients lock in nutrients, which means you're getting more value with every bite. As an added note, when served chicken or pork, remove the skin or rind yourself, as this is where the fat is.

Here's a rundown of what each cooking method entails:

- Poaching: cooking by submerging in liquid

- Baking: cooking method using indirect heat

- Steaming: cooking through heated water vapor

- Broiling: cooking by scorching

- Grilling: cooking method using dry heat

* Sides and snacks

It's common knowledge that when eating out, the most damage to your diet will take place before you even start the actual meal (entrees). This is because this is when snacking happens. From appetizers to that tempting bread basket, people who dine out tend to eat a lot more than they expect.

Unless you're planning on having appetizers as your main course, follow the 3-Bite Rule or skip them completely. And don't go overboard when you get a free helping of starters such as nachos for example. Simple gestures like these are admirable but bad for your diet. If you can't control yourself, you can ask the waiter to remove them from the table (politely of course, or you can ask them not to serve these complementary food items altogether).

As for side dishes, you'll often find a number of them listed down towards the end of a menu (just before the drinks and desserts). For plates that automatically come with side dishes, there's always an option to swap these out. Just ask your waiter.

If your chosen plate comes with creamy or high-calorie side dishes, ask them to replace it with some steamed, roasted, boiled, or baked vegetables for example.

Should you order potatoes and they come with cream, cheese, butter, or bacon, just have these served on the side or not at all. Instead, ask for some chives and salsa. Plain old salt and pepper can also be excellent alternatives.

Again, pay attention when going through the pages of the menu. You'll always find something healthier there. You just have to know what to look for.

* Addressing alcohol

Alcohol is one of those concerns that are often misunderstood, especially when dieting is a part of the discussion. The thing about most restaurant drinks is that, apart from the water, they are laden with sugar. Sodas, juices, cocktails, and the like are laced with unnecessary sugars that kill diets with the snap of a finger.

When it comes to these drinks, they have a high number of empty calories that you are better off consuming in food form. As for alcohol, overindulging in the stuff can affect your reasoning, thereby influencing you to order without much thought or control. For most people, this is enough reason for them to steer clear of it.

But as what was previously mentioned, you shouldn't deprive yourself on an excessive level when you diet because it will only cause you to binge and fall off the ladder. When you choose your alcohol properly, and in the right amounts, it can be something that you can add (without guilt) to your order when you dine out.

The rule of thumb is to limit your alcohol consumption to 150 calories; examples of which are as follows:

- Light Beer (12 ounces)
- Wine (5 ounces, red or white, not the sweet kind)
- Liquor (1.5 ounces, gin, vodka, or tequila)

It's common for people who dine in groups to order by the bottle. In this case, it's a good idea since you'll be able to monitor your intake much easier.

If you're planning on indulging in a multiple-course meal, think about when it would be most proper to take your alcoholic beverage. Just sip on water for the rest of your stay. It's suggested that you take alcohol during the latter part of the meal as doing so will help you control any inhibitions it may lead to, preventing you from uncontrollable ordering and the like.

In addition, don't take alcohol when you haven't eaten anything yet. Drinking on an empty stomach will also lead to inhibitions that you won't appreciate when you're dieting. This is because the alcohol will relax you to the point when you won't think much of what you order or eat when you're out.

So when it comes to alcohol, you can have some but in a limited amount. Remember to save your drink for the latter part of the meal and take it when you've already had something to eat. Enjoy alcohol in moderation and don't let it be the bane of your diet and weight-loss goals.

Chapter 3 Portion Control

Most of the time, you'll find restaurants serving heaping portions of food and this is never good when you're someone who's dieting. Portion control is not something you can expect when you eat out and this is why you have to consider serving sizes when navigating the menu. This is how you can still manage to lose weight even if you eat out on occasion.

Depending on the restaurant, it's possible for the establishment to have fixed servings (one serving size only) for whatever it is they are offering. In this case, go with these visual cues:

- One serving of meat should measure like one deck of cards or the palm of your hand.
- A healthy serving of greens measures in like one open but cupped hand.
- Make a fist. That's how much one serving of fruit or vegetables looks like.
- Ever seen a baseball? That's how much plain baked potato you should have (and supposedly nothing more if you're considering a full serving).
- Four stacked dice is equivalent to one ounce of cheese.
- One serving of salad dressing is pretty much like your thumb.

And then there are those places that offer two to three size options for their meals. In this case, it would be best to go with the smallest serving (usually called a sampler or solo or the so-called "small plate"). This is because their personal or standard serving (usually the second available option) is good enough to share between two people.

So don't think the word "sampler" or "solo" and even "small plate" means that the serving is teeny because more often than not, it's just enough. But don't make the mistake of ordering more than one of these with the reason being that it's indeed a small plate.

Chapter 4 Calorie Counting

If you want to keep up with your diet, lose weight, and still enjoy dining out, you need to start learning how to navigate menus. Previously discussed were the things that you should look for in a particular menu, what to avoid, how to prepare for your night out, the attitude you should have when in the establishment, and how to go about ordering.

But the concept of menu navigation doesn't stop with these. For most people, effective weight loss requires other important practices like counting calories for example. At first, it may seem like an arduous task to undertake. And yes, it can be time consuming. But if you've been counting calories for a while now, expect it to be as simple as reflexes are. At some point, you won't even notice that you're doing it.

When you prepare food at home, the task is easier because you can set up scales and have all the freedom in the world to prepare and measure ingredients without judgment. The same can't be said though when you are out and about. For one, not everyone is into calorie counting and this means that if you attempt to calorie count in a restaurant, you may find yourself on the receiving end of prying eyes, judgmental stares, and a bit of gawking here and there.

It's safe to say that if you're someone who is into counting calories, it will indeed be a challenge to continue doing it when you eat out. But don't be disheartened. Think about it in this manner – when you're counting calories, it's not just about literally measuring ingredients. It's more of tallying the foods that you consume on a daily basis, jotting them down in a handy notebook, or typing them in your mobile phone.

But you might be thinking about how to count calories effectively when it's not you who's preparing the meal. When you eat out, you don't really know how much of a certain ingredient goes into your food and calorie counting isn't really about guessing measurements. Most of the time, chefs themselves don't even measure most of the ingredients that they throw into the mix (like fat and seasonings, all of which add calories to your food).

Given this situation, counting calories may seem like a senseless endeavor when eating out. But do know that there are some tricks that you can use to do this when not eating at home. It all starts with being more mindful of your order. It's basically about knowing what ingredients are in the food you're about to consume.

When you take a look at the menu, chances are you'll find a short description of the meal. This information is enough to give you the bulk of the details that you need to start your calorie counting. When it comes to meat dishes, restaurants also have the tendency to put an ounce measurement of the protein (steaks most especially). As for the other details, you can simply ask your waiter about it (fat, sauces, and other little things).

Unbeknownst to most diners, there are certain health codes per area that make it mandatory for food service establishments to have available food information guides for their clients. So ask your waiter about this as well. If they do have it in-store, chances are you'll be given one of the pamphlets and this will make things even easier on your part.

There is another way to go about it that offers a more private approach to the entire thing. Remember how we talked about doing some research before you do go out? You can apply the same tactic to count calories. As you check the menu prior to your dining date, you can then assess how many calories a plate contains provided that the menu carries a breakdown of the ingredients. Jot down standard serving measurements and simply adjust these later on.

If you're lucky enough to have plans to visit a newer establishment, current diner calorie concerns may mean that you'll receive a menu with the actual calorie counts indicated per meal. You'd usually find these in family restaurants, pubs, and most chain restaurants.

Now this last tip can serve as your last resort or first option (it really depends on how well you trust others with measurements). If you spend enough time looking on the Internet, you'll find a number of websites whose only purpose is to provide calorie counts on different menu items from a wide variety of restaurants across the globe. Especially if the restaurant you're headed off to is someplace known, chances are it'll be listed on at least one of these websites.

Of course, there'll still be instances when you'll be selecting foods without so much as a thought. But a blind decision should not be a detriment to your diet so here's what you should try and do. Before you leave, eat something healthy at home (your pre-game) then choose a healthy option in the restaurant. Instead of jotting down conservative measurements, use the high values on the spectrum. This way, you'll have some wiggle room (a buffer) to work with.

When it comes to weight loss, calorie counting, and addressing limitations on what you eat, your attitude is everything! In the beginning, it's normal to have an odd feeling about things, especially as you start ringing in the numbers with your chosen restaurant dish, but all you have to do to combat this is to focus on a healthy perspective to eating.

Yes, you are dieting. Yes, you want to lose weight. But are certain conditions swaying the way you choose your meals? Don't let excuses like "it's a special celebration" or "this is my reward for going to the gym" be detriments to your goal. Focus on what you want to achieve so as not to underestimate the amount of calories that your chosen food items carry.

Always make wise decisions and never ignore your daily caloric budget. Resources are available to help you with your calorie counting. All you need to do is have the drive or dedication to actually search for them. As they say, if there's a will, then there's a way; and this applies to counting calories when you eat out. The more you get used to the practice, the easier things will be for you the next time you visit your favorite bistro.

Chapter 5 Up Your Foodie Vocabulary – Red Flags

For many people, including those who are actively cutting back and trying to lose weight, eating out isn't something that's easily avoided. On the other hand, eating out will happen more frequently than expected but this is a natural thing; especially for those who are constantly on the go.

As previously mentioned, this is pretty normal and there should be no qualms about it because the issue is not in eating out per se. The problem exists in the failure of most people to navigate menus properly, thereby landing them the wrong meals at the wrong times of day.

The thing about menu navigation is that it helps you avoid excess sugars, carbs, fats, even salt, and other things that can be detrimental to your diet. When you know how to navigate a menu properly, you can choose healthier dishes, allowing you to eat out and still lose weight in the process.

But navigating menus can be more challenging than you think because they are designed to encourage diners to order certain meals. Usually, these meals are high in calories and ingredients that cost the restaurants less money. So even if you're getting a ton of food for what you pay, chances are the restaurant gets a margin that's higher than if you were to order steamed fish or a salad for example.

Foods That are High in Fat

When you're out and are consciously making a healthy food choice, chances are you're not going to be served anything heavily fried. That is if you know how to navigate the menu by steering clear of certain words such as tempura, crusted, battered, golden, breaded, crunchy, or even crispy for example.

Take note of these terms because all of them may not only mean being cooked in a lot of fat but may also have been dredged in flour and coatings that are high in carbohydrates that are easily converted to sugar. And apart from the excess calories, did you know that deep frying removes the foods' natural goodness?

In such a situation, it would be better for you to go with something that has been roaster, grilled, or even baked. These really are some of the terms that you should be looking for when you take a look at a restaurant's menu. Since dishes are usually categorized based on the main protein or ingredients used, focus on these words and you'll be fine.

Foods That Are High in Sugar

If these high-fat foods weren't enough to ruin your diet and make you feel guilty about eating out, you also have a series of foods that are high in sugar to worry about.

A number of restaurants serve sugary meals because they cost less to produce yet encourage diners to order more (as you either can't get enough of it or need something salty to balance the taste out – but regardless of which, you'll end up ordering something else on the menu).

Some of the common terms that restaurants use for these types of food items include glazed, honey-dipped, barbecue or BBQ, teriyaki, and even something as simple as powdered or dusted. These tend to carry a lot of sugar than you'd normally prefer to eat so watch out for them as you go over the menu.

Keep in mind that there are menu items that seem healthy because of the other ingredients that they use like vegetables for example but when added sugars are utilized, they won't enable you to lose weight whilst you enjoy the experience of occasionally eating out. But if there are occasions when you simply can't avoid these food items, don't forget about the 3-Bite Rule.

The same goes for high-carb ingredients. Watch out for pasta, rice, and even starches like white potatoes. Check the menu or ask the waiter if they have whole grain options for the pasta, brown or the mountain variety (minimally processed and un-polished) for the rice, and substitutes for your starch (healthier but equally tasty plantains for example).

Foods That Carry a High Calorie Count

There are also a number of different terms that are used to commonly refer to foods that carry a high number of calories. If you want to eat out and still manage to lose weight then menu items with these words are best avoided – velvety, smothered, rich, loaded, overloaded, creamy, stuffed, cheesy, melted, and gooey.

Upon first glance, these are the kinds of food items most of us would simply love to indulge in but they are some of the worst meals that you can partake in if you're trying to cut back.

As previously mentioned, you should not be swayed by seduc-tive food adjectives. Yes, these words will surely make your mouth water and that is precisely what the restaurant wants to happen, making you order these dishes as a result.

These are perfect examples of comfort foods that can easily transport you back in time but they are also the kinds of meals that can easily transport you to the land of the heavyweights. Even the 3-Bite Rule is not advised in this case as every morsel is usually packed to the punch with calories. Maybe you can sneak a bite but just one.

Foods That Are Actually Good for You

Don't think though that there won't be anything left for you to order after avoiding all of the aforementioned terms (and prob-ably their synonyms). There are other dishes on the menu that deserves your attention and these healthier choices often come with terms such as seasoned, grilled, sautéed, roasted, steamed, spiced, braised, poached, baked, broiled, seared, and rubbed to name a few.

When you see these words on the menu, they usually mean that the food being offered has been prepared and cooked with less fat, sugars, and unnecessary ingredients that add calories without a worry in the world.

Usually, these foods have also been prepared more meticulously than the less healthy options (that's why restaurants encourage diners to order the not-so-healthy fare that are easier and less costly to make) so you are getting more bang for your buck.

Chapter 6 Your Handy Glossary

To make things even easier for you, use this handy term guide the next time you navigate a restaurant menu. Take note of what's good for you, what to avoid, and what best to ask your waiter about.

Green Flag – High Potential of Being Good for You

- Baked – food has been cooked with indirect heat usually without the need for excess fat
- Boiled – food has been cooked by submerging in liquid (most of the time water or stock is used)
- Broiled – similar to baking wherein the food is cooked with indirect heat (includes scorching allowing for quicker cooking)
- Fresh – commonly used by restaurants to refer to raw vegetables
- Grilled – cooked over charcoal, wood, or even a metal plate
- High Fiber – food is high in fiber which aids in digestion and weight loss
- Light – food is low in calories
- Marinated – food is seasoned for a long period of time locking in flavors removing the need for added sugars, sodium, and fat to make meals tasty
- Multi-Grain – food is made with minimally-processed meal (lower in carbohydrate count, higher in fiber levels, more filling)
- Poached – food is cooked over water
- Red Sauce – usually used to refer to rustic tomato sauce (fresh tomatoes, salt, pepper)
- Reduced – when referring to sauces, this means that no thickening agent is used (usually flour or starch) and instead, the sauce has been thickened by simmering it longer
- Roasted – food is cooked with indirect heat with fat usu-

ally allowed to drain away

- Seasoned – refers to restaurant meals where proteins are flavored with natural spices, not thick and high-calorie sauces
- Steamed – food is cooked using water vapor
- Stir-Fried – frying but using high heat (usually in a wok) and a very minute amount of oil (the high heat makes sure that the ingredients don't absorb most of the fat)
- Vegetarian – all ingredients are vegetables
- Vinaigrette – salad dressing consisting of oil and an acid (usually vinegar or citrus fruit like lemon)
- Whole Wheat – minimally-processed meal that's low in carbohydrates, is more filling, and carries a high fiber content

Red Flag - Probably Bad for Your Diet and Weight

- Au Gratin – food has been loaded with cream and topped off with a large amount of cheese
- Barbecue or BBQ – the sauce carries a lot of sugar in different kinds (white, honey, molasses, brown)
- Basted – usually means that thick sauces have been spread over the food before, during, and after cooking
- Battered – food has been dipped into a flour, water, and egg mixture and then deep-fried
- Bearnaise (also called Hollandaise) – a rich, thick, and creamy egg yolk and butter sauce
- Bottomless – this means consume as much as you can and this is not good for weight watchers
- Breaded – the food has been dredged in flour, dipped in eggs, and loaded with breadcrumbs prior to deep frying
- Buttered or Buttery – usually the food is either cooked in or smothered with heaping amounts of butter
- Casserole – similar to a gratin, this commonly involves using heavy cream and cheese
- Cheesy – the cheese added to the food is in large amounts
- Country-Style – this means battered and deep-fried
- Covered – usually means that the food has been indeed covered in velvety sauce

- Creamed or Creamy – the sauce uses heavy cream
- Crispy – the food has been breaded and deep-fried
- Crunchy – also pertains to food being breaded plus deep-fried
- Escalloped – the food, usually a starch like a potato, has been cooked in heavy cream
- Fried/Deep Fried – the food has been cooked by submerging in oil
- Giant – a large serving of food
- Gluten-Free – foods marked as gluten-free comes with added fats and sugars to combat the lack of flavor and to alter the texture to something more appealing
- Loaded – usually pertains to having a large quantity of food or one base ingredient like nachos or bread that's loaded with a number of toppings (with melted cheese and other creamy sauces often included)
- Platter – a selection of different food items in one dish (this is okay if you're going to share the plate)
- Smothered – the food is topped with a heaping serving of rich sauce (usually gravies)
- Stewed – ingredients cooked in heavy sauce (involves the use of thickening agents)
- Stroganoff – the food has been simmered in a rich cream sauce
- Stuffed – a base ingredient is filled with other ingredients (stuffing usually includes bread or breadcrumbs, sometimes even rice and cheese)
- Tempura – the food has been battered and deep-fried
- Value – this is a restaurant trick used to encourage diners to order hefty meals at low prices (this is one of those meals that's cheap to make but comes mostly with batter and fillers instead of actual healthy ingredients)
- Volcano – a volcano overflows and so foods that come with this description usually comes flowing with sauce (commonly cream or cheese-based)
- White Sauce – sauce made primarily with cream

Grey Area – Best to Ask Your Waiter

- Fat-Free – this being good or bad depends on what it pertains to because fat-free cooking is good while a fat-free ingredient is not (because for the latter, sugars and other high-calorie components are used to offset the lack of fat)

Conclusion

Thank you again for downloading this book. Hopefully you learned all about how to properly navigate restaurant menus – from the food to the beverages.

Eating out while dieting and trying to lose weight may not sound like the simplest thing in the world but do know that it's indeed possible. All you really have to do is allot a reasonable amount of time to research and reading.

Keep in mind that when you decide to eat out, your first challenge won't be the food that's going to be served but the menu. The way you use the menu can make a big difference in how your diet will pan out.

There are ways for you to navigate menus that will not only help you find healthy food options but find enough food to order ensuring that your dining experience will be a memorable one. This is because when you're dieting, putting too many restrictions on what you can and can't consume can be detrimental to the process.

This way, by knowing which foods are good to order, you'll be able to indulge in flavorful meals without the guilt in your stomach and added pounds on the scale.

Do your research before you head out. The Internet is your oyster so use it to your advantage. There are plenty of useful information, reviews, calorie quantifications, and the like, online. Find these information and make choosing what to order easier on your part.

Also read the descriptions on food items in a menu. They are there for a reason. If you need more assistance then don't be afraid to ask the waiter. Again, they are there to help you out. And if you find something on menus that you feel won't work with your diet, politely ask the chef to prepare things your way (if possible).

These days, more and more restaurants are readily accommodating the specific dietary requirements of their clients so chances are they'll be prepared to manage certain requests without fail.

Count calories and portions even when you're out. Look for keywords in the menu and don't let taste bud-tantalizing words seduce you. Whenever you're looking at the menu, don't fall for sweet words. Always think "healthy" and watch out for terms such as smothered, heaping, enveloped, rich, and so on and so forth.

Use categories (especially for beverages) to your advantage. Use them to narrow down your options especially if you're faced with quite a lengthy menu. You know what your diet calls for so use these categories to make more informed decisions on whatever it is you'll be ordering, food or drink. And of course, spend time understanding the contents of this book and don't find it extra to do more research on the topic at hand.

If at first you don't succeed, try and try again. And don't be disheartened if you experience some difficulty at first as this is quite normal. The more you engage in these tactics to navigate menus and eat out while still being able to lose weight, the more natural everything will feel the next time you eat out with friends or family.

The next step is to take what you've learned and apply them in a real-life setting. Give yourself time to adjust, make alterations to your system, and check out which strategies work for you or not. In this case, it's all about what works best for you and no one else.

Hopefully you have learned a lot from this book and realize that you can enjoy the occasional restaurant experience without gaining back pounds you've lost dieting.

Finally, if you enjoyed this book, then I'd like to ask you for a favor, would you be kind enough to leave a review for this book on the site where you purchased it, or on Amazon? It'd be greatly appreciated!

The Online Trainers

Is a business providing professional fitness programs and advise at an affordable rate.

Check out my blog, fitness programs, and store at theonline-trainers.com

www.ingramcontent.com/pod-product-compliance
Lightning Source LLC
Chambersburg PA
CBHW031334290526
45784CB00014B/2715